"With immense poetic resources, and weaving together the fabric of her life into a great tapestry, Bahar Orang reflects on beauty in terms of medical identity, love, race, and art. Variably paced, with a vibrant feminist subjectivity, Orang's debut is worthy of its subject, devising 'new shapes for intimacy, new words for care.' An incredible work."

SHANE NEILSON, AUTHOR OF *NEW BRUNSWICK*

Where Things Touch

A MEDITATION ON BEAUTY

Bahar Orang

Essais Series No. 10

Book*hug Press
TORONTO

FIRST EDITION
copyright © 2020 by Bahar Orang
ALL RIGHTS RESERVED

Library and Archives Canada Cataloguing in Publication

Title: Where things touch : a meditation on beauty / Bahar Orang.
Names: Orang, Bahar, 1992– author.
Series: Essais (Toronto, Ont.) ; no. 10.
Description: Series statement: Essais series ; 10 | A poetically
influenced essay.
Identifiers: Canadiana (print) 20200159402 | Canadiana (ebook)
    20200160575 | ISBN 9781771665698 (softcover)
    ISBN 9781771665704 (HTML) | ISBN 9781771665711 (PDF)
    ISBN 9781771665728 (Kindle)
Classification: LCC PS8629.R36 W54 2020 | DDC C814/.6—DC23

Printed in Canada

The production of this book was made possible through the generous
assistance of the Canada Council for the Arts and the Ontario Arts
Council. Book*hug Press also acknowledges the support of the
Government of Canada through the Canada Book Fund and the
Government of Ontario through the Ontario Book Publishing Tax
Credit and the Ontario Book Fund.

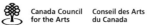

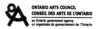
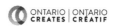

Book*hug Press acknowledges that the land on which we operate
is the traditional territory of many nations, including the Mississaugas
of the Credit, the Anishnabeg, the Chippewa, the Haudenosaunee
and the Wendat peoples. We recognize the enduring presence of many
diverse First Nations, Inuit and Métis peoples and are grateful for
the opportunity to meet and work on this territory.

For M

[   ]

Perhaps my project began when Solmaz Sharif wrote

My life can pass like this
Waiting for beauty

[   ]

Perhaps my writing, here, is the articulation of a
series of ruptures—all the times I appeared to
be waiting but was actually searching. My search has
changed, though, because I hardly know anymore
whether I can even articulate that aporia that is beauty,
or if it even wishes to be expressed at all.

[   ]

And then there is your beauty, a beauty that appears
to me rather like the sun, rather like the moon.

[   ]

And by this I mean that every lock of curly black hair
extends from its root, reaching beyond itself, light
and messy and stubborn. And we might say you have
an olive complexion, a chromatic kind of fairness
that glows into the night.

[   ]

And there is, somehow, the presence of beauty between
us. A beauty that offers more than its playful glimmer;
a beauty that opens its arms to us, considers stillness as
its impermanent home. We could not rush to capture
that beauty, such an impulse would be its opposite.

[   ]

But here I am idealizing beauty, purifying beauty,
as though it's not wrapped up in the mess of desire
and regret in which we live, as though beauty does
not already reside in a home of fragmented language
and memory.

[   ]

Because your ex, the person you dated before me,
won't stop calling you. You say you once found them
beautiful. You say this with your arm leaning against
the windowsill, next to a potted purple hyacinth, a
sombol, not quite in bloom, that lives free from
doubt or withholding, that knows just what it needs,
the sun.

[   ]

But before I go any further, I have this to offer,
a touchstone:

There's a strangeness, for sure, but a sense of
recognition, too—the moving image is like
something that's escaped from the fissures of my
own heart. I guess perhaps a wistfulness, but only
the wistfulness of everyday life, the poet's feeling
that all of us feel all the time. And a sunset, very
slight, casting a yellowish glow over the street,
small circles of light reflecting from the car's
windows; we watch from a car driving behind two
men on a motorbike, riding down the streets of
Tehran, one man trying to steady a bouquet of
crooked pink flowers and their too-long green stems.

The flowers might be dahlias, *kokab*. It's the final
scene of Kiarostami's film *Close-Up*, and we've
arrived, I'm sure, at one definition of beauty —
a sort of lighthouse, somewhere to start.

[   ]

I'm sitting in a psychiatry clinic, on my first rotation
as a medical student. I wanted to start with psychiatry
because the sight of blood still makes me uneasy.
It's too much redness at once, a colour too arresting,
too unambiguous, without intimation or forethought.
I can't find the words, there are no words, really,
for a red that symbolizes nothing, that is only the
thing itself. Red for red's sake.

[   ]

Instead of words for red, I have images. In particular,
the moving image of the artist Ana Mendieta: her
hands and arms coated with blood, pressing herself,
her arched body, against white sheets of paper, and

then dragging the red, a slow descent, down the wall
to the ground.

[ ]

This piece, *Body Tracks*, is not an abbreviation of the body,
not a memory, not an imprint, neither imitation nor
abstraction, but a new fragment of self, in which the
palpable body—its bone, skin, and sinew—cannot be
repressed or destroyed. Blood, or body tracks, seems
to efface the limits of the body, and even in witness,
or in spectatorship, we become linked to that body,
in all its utter and abject materiality.

[ ]

Every colour is a kind of beauty, and Mendieta's red
might insist on life, after all, on an embodied life,
where only things felt can be known, can be beauty.

[ ]

Another red thing: poppies, *khash khash*. Poppies are not meant to be potted, they can never be kept by florists, they are wildflowers that resist any other kind of life. What happens to beauty when it's removed from its own dirt? If you pick a poppy, it withers within the hour. How simple a practice, then, to let flower, let flower, smelling its own earth.

[   ]

The poet Sohrab Sepehri: *As long as the poppies bloom, life must be lived.* I'll come to think of this line many times through the long and strange months of my training, imagining a poppy field at night, with quiet as the language and abundance the only course.

[   ]

There's a tall doctor sitting before me, removing an invisible fleck of dust from his suit. We're discussing a pregnant young patient whom we just met. He insists: this woman has borderline personality disorder. Borderline patients, he says, are afflicted with "chronic

feelings of emptiness," with "unstable relationships,"
with "a shifting sense of self."

[ ]

It's strange to sift through his language—sometimes
they are borderline people, other times they have
a borderline diagnosis, and still other times they
have borderline traits. Which is it? Are they their
personality or do they contain a personality? What is
the structure of personality? This seems essential
to know, because how else can we trace the borders
that are dashed or wrecked, or know what's swelling
at some seam? And how to test the hypothesis that
personality, or person, should be an integer, fixed
and immovable?

[ ]

I take notes as he speaks, but remain expressionless,
resisting his gestures that beckon me to mimic,
or share in, or forgive him for his exasperation,
his amusement, his dismissiveness of our patient.

He will later write in my evaluation: *you appear very serious and stoic, and this will be misconstrued by patients.*

[   ]

At this clinic, the psychiatrists can be hesitant to take on so-called borderline patients. Of course, most of the borderline diagnoses are women, and the hesitant doctors are men. I try to suggest this obvious pattern to my supervising physician, and a knowing look crosses his face, like suddenly he has me figured out.

[   ]

But really, I'm thinking only of your ex-lover, another so-called borderline person, whose pain has become so present in our lives that I, too, am taken up by it, caring, by accident, for them, in spite of myself.

[   ]

Psychiatrists might name such a response to a patient as countertransference, an experience to acknowledge and keep in check. I admit, it's messy: a patient, someone I might one day treat, reminds me of my lover's ex-lover. But here, in my uncertainty and discomfort, where categories reveal their fallibility, I might enter the third space: neither hospital nor home, neither clinic nor street, but an unnamed, unclaimed place of possibility, where I might imagine new shapes for intimacy, new words for care.

[   ]

Beauty must be in conversation with care—there can be no alternative for me! So when I say beauty, I mean the slow approach of alive things, meeting each other in all their complexity and longing.

[   ]

The doctor talks drugs, but it's raining now and getting dark outside. The sound of the rain, a rhythm without a cause, permits me to think of other things. What are the

borders of care? Can we speak of borders even as we
speak of entanglement? The doctor turns on the light,
and I think of how it feels to write in the dark, how the
words on the page become indiscernible, shapeless,
the notebook itself barely different than my lap, meaning
is here somewhere, unreadable, probably untenable.

[　]

I write letters to you in the dark, hoping my latent
desires, which I describe so unsuccessfully in the light,
can look like beauty in the dark, not for the purpose
of intelligibility, just to be apprehended as singular
and strange.

[　]

Can we imagine language as a sort of border of care?
In which case my efforts here to describe beauty are
acts of love. Though it's a project with its own perils,
sometimes language is only omission.

[　]

Not to mention that there are days when beauty is as borderless as the sea, an entity that evokes without recoil, that opens, only opens. What is our relationship to that sea? The sea whose large hands sweep away whatever footprints we leave in the sand, whose blue displaces me from any centre.

[   ]

Artist and writer Etel Adnan: *to look at the sea is to become what one is*. The sea, if you allow it, settles the itinerancy of the human heart, the heart that flits about, lovesick, trying to accumulate meaning from this thing or that thing, travelling from here to there, running from tedium, mistaking tumult for freedom. The sea is like the final poem, and the performance of looking a never-ending feat. Looking is freedom, looking to the sea, becoming what one is, a revelation of beauty.

[   ]

A sort of looking at the sea: Adnan's landscape paintings, where the horizon is sometimes shifted, sometimes even absent, where colours are so expressive that you want to reach out and touch them. Blue suns, pink waters, slightly slant lines, all stillness. I don't know. For me, these paintings say solitude, a radical solitude, with all their frankness and their silence. At the same time, the sun is dependent on the mountain is dependent on the sea; one thing becomes the other, in no linear order, together and apart.

[   ]

It is one effect of beauty to soften contradiction; indeed, to offer another language where there is no contradiction to begin with, where a mountain's solitude is necessary for its intimacy with the sun, where a viewer's solitude brings them closer to the art, allowing the art to become a sentient, social being of its own.

[   ]

Another look at the sea: Sappho, emerging. Some say she came from the sea, another wave, and I like to

think of her this way, a glistening body in stride,
the only possible rupture for an unchanging ocean.

[ ]

Sappho's poems, the physical objects that they are,
decaying fragments, yellow papyrus in jagged shapes,
are experiments of beauty in their own right. Poems
are not pure, they, too, are subject to ruination by
bacteria, by water, by soil, by wind, and by creature.
But it's an aesthetics, an aesthetics of ruination,
the poems are returned to us anew, and we are in
conversation with the particles of the earth.

[ ]

What I mean to say is this: Sappho is like a vector
of desire, she has cracked the mystery of desire, and
here we are in her wake, trying, with all the materials
available to us, to get at that immensity, that
impossibility that is desire, that is sometimes beauty.

[ ]

Desire, we often think, is about something lacking, about wanting, filling a hole. Desire, we might say at first, is in the empty spaces of Sappho's poem-pieces. But what of desire as repetition, same and different, layers overlapping and shifting; Sappho's poems whole as they are, but with an infinite number of possible relations with any reader, any strange molecule. And beauty here, in each engagement.

[   ]

We met in July in a loud bar in the village. You were dancing ecstatic, jeans and white T-shirt like skin. I don't remember first touch or first kiss, only my own apprehension, a shyness I tried to project as coyness, as your small hips, small shoulders, moved into the space between us, words giving way, sensation the only thing left.

[   ]

When I learned that you're writing a dissertation on freedom, I wondered about the logic between freedom

and beauty; perhaps all free things are not necessarily
beauty, but I suspect that all things of beauty are
necessarily free.

[   ]

The day after our first meeting, it was still summer,
warm sunrise, a fan whirring nearby,
but otherwise it was stillness.
I can't say I stayed for very long,
I saw your face again in the sunlight
and it was half sleeping, half hanging pothos plant,
I thought of spending the whole day with you
until it could be evening again
and we might sit on the porch,
cold beers and paperbacks,
but I couldn't rearrange you any better even if I tried
an improvised picture,
how the hair fell, how the sweat fell,
the rhythm of your breathing,
covers thrown away, sheets strewn,
so I left you in your stillness, your morning,
as one does for sleeping animals.

[   ]

I was equally in love with you, with the window,
the fan, the possible paperbacks, and the green pothos
I imagined to be the form of your body. I was in love
with the ecosystem of where we were, and I only hoped
it could love me back. These are the queer love stories
that interest me, encounters of beauty between
sunlight and pillow—between summer and stillness.

[   ]

I revise: beautiful things are not necessarily free;
instead, beauty beckons freedom, approaches it,
tastes and remembers it, reaching for freedom with
tendrils asymmetric and awake.

[   ]

At the hospital, still during my first few months of
training, I discuss the size of a toddler's stools with
her father. Are they the width of a nickel? A quarter?
The child is severely constipated and in great pain.
He shakes his head, unsure, at a loss. We try laxatives
and dietary changes, but nothing works. He tells us

about her fraught relationship to her bowels. She hates having her diaper changed, she hates all our clinical exams, and most of all she will hate having an enema, which seems to be the only remaining option. The pediatrician explains that the procedure will be quick, she is unlikely to remember it, and afterwards she'll feel relief.

[ ]

Memory tends to live in provisional places—under fingernails, between creases of the palm, where the spine curves, our unpredictable behaviours, our predictable behaviours, the proximity we permit our lovers, timbre and tone, in the skin and how it folds, what we consider beautiful, what seems like a choice but is not, what seems like an accident but is not, how certain meetings feel like anguish and others like a wharf, a wharf facing some other possibility. Our young patient might feel relief, but how and what she remembers, the effect of the memory, this part is less certain.

[ ]

When I go to see her in the early morning before the procedure, I don't know how to speak to what's about to happen, how to express things as questions, how to include her. Her father comes into the room and cradles her against his chest. I feel frozen with anxiety and astonishment, defenceless against the staggering vulnerabilities and dependencies of our little bodies. How we come into being in relation to each other, how swiftly we can slip into violence, how we're all bound up in this fleshy project, love.

[   ]

I asked for beauty, and among bodies in pain, illusions of irreproachability, between linoleum floors and white lights is where I ended up.

[   ]

I might return now to Solmaz Sharif's poem "Beauty," another part, where she writes:

You asked for beauty, and one morning, a small blue
eggshell on the stoop, shattered
open, its contents gone
Likely eaten

[   ]

Which is beauty? The contents eaten, that which
is gone, a mystery? Or the eggshell's fragments,
shattered open, their blue, their dispersal? Or: does
asking for beauty eat beauty, is asking for beauty
a violence to beauty? Does she mean that beauty will
not show up on a stoop, whole, that beauty haunts us,
beauty's bird like a ghost, leaving only pieces behind?

[   ]

But "Beauty" did show up on my stoop, with words
beautiful, addressing me, the poem itself an eggshell
shattered open, pointing to the unsayable.

[   ]

How does one resolve oneself to the condition of unsayability? How does one accept that language is painful, that the practice of articulating by word, whether to express beauty or care, is a blemish on the page, a crack in the silence, a fragment working to recuperate all that exceeds it?

[   ]

Having a drink with you, I am caught between the impulse to say so many things, everything, and to say nothing at all, to treat our moment with diligence. At the very least, I want to invent a new language to address you, something that better expresses my ambivalence, but don't get me wrong, the ambivalence is a pleasurable one. I want a new language, our secret, but the old words keep slipping in. I can neither escape nor resist them.

[   ]

What if language were to remember how fragile it is, and how flawed? Words that are beautiful position themselves as Mary Oliver's lilies:

They rise and fall
in the edge of the wind,
and have no shelter
from the tongues of the cattle

[   ]

These are flowers that understand their home is the
mouth of another creature, just as words belong
where they, too, can rise and fall—that is, in relation
to what lives around them: the words that are their
neighbours, the readers who consider them, and all
the landscapes that allow them to exist.

[   ]

Before, I was sure I would spend the better part of my
time studying words, reading and writing, learning
beauty, looking to flowers. But I went to medical school
instead, and medicine, with all the shit, blood, and guts,
does not wear beauty on its sleeve.

[   ]

An early memory of trying for beauty: a short story
I wrote at age ten, wherein a young boy, Idlum, loses
his mother and walks every day to a wide-open field
to share his memories of her with a wide-open sky.
He addresses the sky as "sky," and refers to "sky" as his
best friend. After this story, for a while, my writing
always featured an Anne or a Jane, in love with a
Darcy or George. The borders of my imaginary blunted
any beauty, and I never finished a story. I was too bored
to carry on.

[   ]

Another time I tried for beauty: the old desk I found
for you. Its oak is discoloured, and the previous owner
has carved her initials on its face, but it's a living thing
in the room, with its many textures and troughs,
offering itself for the work, the work of thinking and
writing, the work of curiosity and consideration.
I stack three books at its corner, tape a photograph
to the wall, put three yellow tulips, *laleh*, in a vase,
and gently flip open some of their petals.

[   ]

Now, when I say beauty, I could mean flowers, and
how they desire, or how I desire them. Flowers are so
continuous with their environments, so reliant on
everything around them—sunlight, insects, rain—
that we might forget how tulips, *laleh*,
rise suddenly,
a rush of blood,
totally free.

[   ]

Beauty, like memory, can only be defined
provisionally. There is no complete essay to write
on beauty, no final word, no quintessential image.
Please understand, beauty is not a problem to be
solved; beauty is not a question to be answered;
beauty denies enclosure or straightforwardness.
Beauty is something opening, and if you are lucky,
the thing opening is you, your body, your palms
and your feet, so you are more surface to press
against the earth.

[   ]

We're walking quickly down a busy street at night, excited by our conversation, our hands bump into each other until finally you grab mine; every so often I trace my finger up the side of your arm before letting my hand fall back into yours, I glance up sometimes to admire your profile, your skin, the wind is warm, few things are better than a warm wind, we wander in and out of shops, hardly noticing them, all our cells laughing, the whole of our skin trembling.

[   ]

Detachment and coolness, my usual games, are not possible between us.

[   ]

I ask more about your ex, and you tell me how they found you so smart, so beautiful, so interesting. You tell me how they admitted to a type: Middle Eastern lovers. Back then, you say, you didn't mind this so much, and maybe even felt more special and loved for

it. They were an art history student, and I perform
indignance, pointing out something I consider Art
History 101: *the limitations of Orientalism are the
limitations that follow upon disregarding, essentializing,
denuding the humanity of another culture, people.* You
shrug, I shrug back.

[   ]

We talk about ethics. I offer that every manner of
loving is an experiment, that the only way to love
is by trial and error. But there are stakes for those
errors. Each trial is a risky game, a continual
dispossession of ourselves for another. *With* another,
you suggest.

[   ]

Secretly, I am thinking only of beauty, hesitant to
reveal that to you yet. What kinds of beauty did you
see in each other? Philosopher Elaine Scarry writes,
Beauty always takes place in the particular, and how
particular you are, how very singularly odd and

attractive, appearing in my life without problem or precedent. Nothing has been more erotic than your bumpy, callused hands carrying a small bouquet of calla lilies, *gole sheypoori*, wrapped in newspaper, placing them gently into an empty wine bottle later that night.

[   ]

One possible ethics of loving: Sappho's broken poems, and how they allow their reader to look away and return, look away and return. The poems offer room for the weight of a reader's own body—a triangular romance between Sappho, space, and self. To engage ethically with Sappho's poems is to love fragments, to love in fragments, with no totalizing category, no interest in a lost whole, no disdain for flaws. Such an encounter between lovers is to bring together only the honest pieces that we are, to know indeterminacy as precious.

[   ]

A fragment from Sappho:

]
]*nor*
]*desire*
]*but all at once*
]*blossom*
]*desire*
]*took delight*

[   ]

Beauty, I imagine, is desire twice, is all at once, is delight,
the open bracket, something asking to be touched.

[   ]

Eventually I admit to you my preoccupation with
beauty, only to realize how little I really have to say
about it. Why does beauty interest me? It's more than
an interest, I offer. Beauty guides me. There are so
few serious ideas I can stay with if there is no
engagement with beauty. There are so few things I

can write about if beauty is not at the heart. Beauty governs me. No, it's not an obsession. No, it's not just a project. Well, maybe it is. A project that is my life.

[   ]

Louise Glück, in her poem "The Red Poppy," writes: *I speak because I am shattered.* Beauty shatters, makes fragments from anything, turns body to debris. But it's a shattering through which speaking becomes possible. In Glück's poem, the speaker is a poppy, a fragment of the universe, a fragment among fragments, not entirely discrete but still free, free at the edge of her own particular location, her own particular longing.

[   ]

Actually, "The Red Poppy" was recommended to me by a patient who suggests it when I tell her I am writing a piece on beauty, maybe about flowers. She's a woman close to her death, and who had at one point been an English teacher. She can't remember the name of the poem, and only recites to me how it starts:

The great thing
is not having
a mind. Feelings:
oh, I have those.

[   ]

Something in me says that I can't share the poem with
the physicians I'm working with, that they'd have no
interest in considering a poppy's subjectivity,
especially a subjectivity made by feeling rather than
by mind. I'll learn, soon enough, that it's not an
entirely accurate assumption on my part, that many
physicians, especially trainees, share my desire to
think about beauty instead of suffering, or rather,
to integrate beauty into reflections on suffering.
I'll learn that many of us already understand,
instinctively, that in any place of suffering there are
islands of beauty. And not sentimentality, not cliché—
beauty. All of us in any clinic or hospital, patients
and caregivers—we are starved for it, beauty.

[   ]

I invite you to stay with me for four weeks in a tiny
southwestern town where I am to complete another
clinical rotation in pediatrics. It's January now, and
there is very little to do in this town. But you can use
the large space I am renting out and spend the days
working on your thesis. In the evenings we can read
next to each other, watch movies, make large dinners.
On the weekends we'll walk along a nearby beach,
let the cold wind of the water jolt us awake.

[   ]

Between patients, during my lunch hour, we write
back and forth about beauty. No, you say, that which
is just or is good sometimes happens to be beautiful.
No, I respond, beauty runs through nearly all that
is just or is good. You ask: So we should follow beauty
to justice or goodness? I respond: No, it only comes to
be in reflection, or in experience, moment to moment—
So why dwell on it at all?
For this question, I still have no good or satisfying
answer. Instead, I ask back: Do you think writing on
beauty makes the writing beautiful?

(I imagine your skeptical face, looking through me,
amused at the insecurity I try to mask as vanity.)

[   ]

At night, you breathe in my bare stomach,
flip me over, and ask,
How badly do you want it?
(As bad as a most diffuse rain, who,
despite its shreddedness,
remembers the ocean,
yes, knows itself still
mostly as ocean.)

[   ]

I learn how many ways there are to spell home:
your foot, your shoe, the lamp, the chair, creases
in paper, unmade beds, our night.

[   ]

Is beauty simply home? But with this question I might just be moving from one indeterminate question to another, from one plural place to another, from one lesson in the sacred possibility of difference to another.

[   ]

That being said, it seems an easy way out, an uninteresting way out, and probably a dangerous way out, to suggest that beauty is only subjective, with a limitless number of possible meanings. Because some meanings are trite and others are violent, so there must be something left to say with a good degree of certainty.

[   ]

I ask you whether beauty is just another word for home and you describe an idea of modal music, where each key has a note that names the key and sounds maybe like home. When you play progressions of other notes in the key, the home-note is where the ear always feels compelled to return. And when you play other keys altogether, there is tension,

because the ear longs for resolution, to return to
the note, home.

[   ]

Whatever beauty is, I know it has little to do with
origins or symmetry. But something here still rings
true: it's the ear in longing, I think, but longing is just
our word for knowing—knowing what? Knowing that
it's all happening together at the same time: the
return home, the release from home, the home-note
as the only note played again and again. Because our
universe is far too complex, too textured, for a music
where every possible iteration does not happen at
once, somewhere near and beyond our ears.

[   ]

Partway through our winter, you get sick with a cough
and a runny nose. I come home to see you curled up
on the couch, breathing noisily, and I am suddenly
filled with a frank tenderness. I can immediately
name it as tenderness, and it is as familiar to me as

something I might have felt every day for all my life. I suggest that this, too, is an experience of beauty. Also our greeting, my hand through your hair before I go to the kitchen to put on some hot water.

[   ]

We return to the city, and you tell me that you will have coffee with the ex. On the day of your meeting, I go to a Yoko Ono exhibit at the Gardiner. In her work *MendPiece*, Ono instructs viewers: *Take me to the farthest place in our planet by extending the line.* She offers materials for our play: white gallery walls, a hammer, nails, paper, pencils, glue, string, broken pieces of pottery. I put a nail into the wall, tie my string around it, and attach its other end some three metres away to another crooked nail that someone has put in before me.

[   ]

You meet me at the museum and tell me about how the ex returned some of your old records, how they

expressed an interest in friendship. They also gave
you a gift: a small, golden sarcophagus pendant.
You're not sure what to do with it. I hand you a nail,
some string, and a ceramic shard the shape of your
lips. I observe your lips in many places now.

[   ]

The pendant strikes me as a racist object, but you
say you'll keep it. I feel that you'd be keeping a
ghost, as perhaps I, too, would do if the gift had
been for me from an ex-lover, whose ghosts,
I suppose, are also the ghosts of our past selves,
sweetbitter pieces we both love and despise,
ghosts we want to forget or excise. I wonder if
we'd do better to treat our ghosts with some
kindness for the imperfect, trembling species
they are.

[   ]

I hang another fragment to the wall and look around
the large room, where string and nail make complex

configurations, white ceramic parts floating, *a poetics of the whole fragment.*

[　]

I think we must be these ceramic bodies, these shattered pieces hanging from lines of desire, desire that feels at once like affliction and freedom, like beauty and pain. Suddenly I realize that beauty is at times inextricable from pain, that beauty is nothing if not an essential detail of relation, of entanglement, and we are so fragile as we edge nearer and nearer to each other, inhabiting that third space, inhabiting a perpetual state of vulnerability, wavering between wreckage and repair.

[　]

Third spaces as gaps, holes, crevices and cracks, misshapen flowers, misshapen artworks, not emptiness, not saturation, certain embraces, certain encounters, some colours, some ghosts, bewilderment, places of uncertainty, places of mystery, handwritten

notes for a possible poem—that is, the first impulse
to testify against fixity, against the fallacy of a closed
and unchangeable world.

[   ]

Medical dictionaries define "third space" as *the
non-functional area between cells that when filled with
fluid, become dangerous.* And "third-spacing," as
physicians call it, is highly concerning in the
biomedical sense—when the heart, lungs,
or abdomen become flooded. But in a poetic or
aesthetic mode, third-spacing is like a sidestep,
a discernment or an improvisation, straying from
the established path to follow beauty into
unknowingness.

[   ]

There is one particular silueta by Ana Mendieta,
Untitled, from her *Silueta Series*, made in Mexico,
where the silueta is comprised of small red flowers,
lying at the coast in the sand, inches away from water.

Slow waves brush up against the silueta's untidy
borders, a few flowers already scattered along
the ocean's foamy edge, pressed into the fissures
of sea rocks. The body of this piece is made only of
third space, all of it about to be filled with fluid,
so precarious, and yet not at all as it returns, finally,
to the place from which it came, the earth.

[   ]

Though Mendieta has placed the flowers self-consciously,
into a particular shape, beauty is a matter of chance,
too, as the shape plays with the waves in an unscripted
manner, waves that are unpredictable, that act of their
own unmediated will. Mendieta relies on this relation
of effacement: the waves will disperse her flowers,
but she can't know precisely when or how. I think
of Simone Weil, who describes beauty as *the harmony
of chance and good*. The chance: the spontaneities,
the creative impulses, of the sea. The good: the
freedom of a body pressed into the sand, an artist
reckoning, an artist slipping away.

[   ]

By beauty, then, I mean slippage, I mean untetherment;
I mean letting go, letting go of certainty, of expectation;
I mean the notes for the poem, the poem that cannot
otherwise be expressed; I mean the image reflected
briefly in the mirror, in your eyes, your good brown
eyes that move me, in spite of myself, into sentimentality,
that embarrassing mode; I mean the image reflected
in the water, ocean as artist, body as subject, tides
moving to their own intuition.

[   ]

Is beauty the moment of tension between two or
more parts, where friction is sweet, things touch,
and the possibility of togetherness slips through the
poet's fingers?

[   ]

Aesthetic experience is like that, it slips through us.
And although our *aesthetic judgments are always
impure*, standing on the balcony, the tiniest balcony in
the whole city, a balcony that feels nonetheless like a

castle, the winter is breaking, the days are longer, the
outside air has a new texture now, something balmy,
something falling away, and I'm granted meaning,
or is it pleasure, a distance and a closeness at once, I'm
both lover and beloved, I face a setting sun, a rustling
in my body, things clearer for the moment.

[　]

Beauty is the pink twilight hours of lying in bed with
you, laid bare of language or totality, curled open like
orange blossoms of springtime, *baharnarenj*, delivered
finally, attentive and wild.

[　]

I'm in the OR, watching as the obstetrician draws an
incision with a scalpel across the pregnant woman's
bikini line, and it figures like the line through a word
that's not quite right. Or Derrida's writing *sous rature*,
which Spivak translates as *under erasure*. Spivak goes
on: *this is to write a word, cross it out, and then print
both word and deletion.*

Since the word is inaccurate, it is crossed out.
Since it is necessary, it remains legible.

[   ]

The doctor questions me on the anatomy of the woman's
insides, and words fail me. I know the answer! But
I'm sputtering at the sight of blood—a rising in my belly
for which there are few words. To see a person open
on an operating table, for this, words are a wave moving
along an infinite asymptote.

[   ]

Neither my degree in English Literature nor my degree
in Comparative Literature compelled me to read, with
any real openness or incisiveness, Derrida, or Deleuze,
or whatever else we might traditionally call Philosophy
or Critical Theory or otherwise. I suppose I was a bad
student, skimming through my readings, silent in
class—equal parts bored and intimidated—writing
with conviction only as needed. There were times I felt
inspired, and I was thoughtful or creative—usually

under the mentorship of a teacher who had done away
with the canon, who, in one broad stroke, freed their
students from any notion of a compulsory reading list. I
learned to think and write through a curious
kaleidoscope of things: comics and poems, writing by
artists who never went to art school, children's books,
portraits of Frida Kahlo—and so on.

[   ]

Even lovers have tried to impress upon me the
importance of reading Hegel or Heidegger, lovers
who have declared my sheepish disinterest a
symptom of a modern, shallow throng. In one case, I
was advised to be permanently suspicious of beauty.
How unnerving, then, all the times this same lover
remarked that I was beautiful.

[   ]

Meanwhile, there's a hypothesis in medicine: reading,
a word unconsidered and unqualified, will make you a
more empathetic and humane doctor. Except I have

known students and scholars who, despite all their literary cunning and writerly prowess, seem to know little about things like compassion. I have known readers, voracious readers who, in reading, simply reinforce their own small-minded beliefs—readers who find, by reading, new logics and arguments for those beliefs. Readers with little interest in recovering beauty, whose queer is not concerned with flowers.

[ ]

And the poet Forough Farrokhzad, who said: *I believe in being a poet in all moments of life. Being a poet means being human. I know some poets whose daily behaviour has nothing to do with their poetry.* Again, how essential to rescue poetry from purity, and to know, in turn, that beauty is as varied and polysemic as desire; I suppose I'm confusing terms here, but poetry, beauty, desire—they are impossible to disentangle, and I feel deeply invested in the possibilities of their entanglement. What emerges from such a mess? Pain, surely. Freedom, maybe. When desire undoes you, when your aching parts open and glisten like gossamer, when poems of beauty fill you with stillness touched by longing, longing touched by stillness,

when you traverse your own pain, its edges like
pleasure, freedom conceivable.

[   ]

There is not a book in this world that, upon simply
being read, will make you a better doctor or person.
And we know that's especially true about writing of
the canon, any canon. But I'm returning now to
Of Grammatology, reading it in the clinic, after class,
between patients. I suppose I was moved by the story
of Spivak—a young scholar who came across Derrida's
text in French, translated it into English, and her
translation, framed by her book-length introduction,
was enormously successful, became canon.

[   ]

Despite all my years of resistance, Spivak digs a little
hole in my palm, into which I imagine a Derrida smugly
falling. But so embedded am I in the traditions and
philosophies of the Western world that I can hardly trust
myself when suddenly I see something anew and it's

beautiful. White people cite white people into banality
and violence, and I've been known to follow, falling for
their displays of liberal politics, for their reassurance
that, yes, Hegel matters less now, but White is still the
moniker of sophistication, intellect, poetry, and beauty.
And I feel like a cliché, a phony, a shape of imagination
itself, as I stand there in Farokhzad's wind, *the wind will
carry us*—breathing in dreams of Sepehri's flowers,
of orange blossoms I've never really known.

[   ]

The pregnant woman is awake for her C-section. She
lies flat on her back with a cloth screen hanging down
at her chest. This way, she can't see what's happening at
the level of her abdomen, where we cut through skin,
fatty layer, fascia, muscle, peritoneum, and then uterus.
It's a startling, nearly unfathomable sight: the woman is
behind the screen, talking nervously with her husband,
and on the other side, an OB, several nurses, and I are
opening her up, blood flowing, organs and slimy bits
protruding. And at the end of the dig: baby! The lower
half of the woman's body is numb, but she feels
pressure as our intention gets deeper and the digging
gets harder. It's not a terribly controlled or clean

surgery—the surgeon wrestles, hard, with the uterus to reach baby, blood spills freely, and amniotic fluid shoots out playfully as everyone chortles and steps back.

[   ]

I peek behind the curtain, and the woman's husband is stroking her cheek, repeating IloveyouIloveyou. I think of you and the first time I thought to utter "I love you," and the very small poem I wrote to that effect:

well we don't want to say *I love you*
it might be too easy, too much
instead we get inside the words,
to a naked centre,
peeling off their paper,
open in my hand, soft bones,
what a lovely,
aching game it is:
finding all the ways to say
what you mean to me

(everything).

[   ]

It was another crossing-out, I suppose — a loving *sous rature*.

[ ]

Spivak explains in an interview: *That's what deconstruction is about, right? It's not just destruction. It's also construction. It's critical intimacy, not critical distance. So you actually speak from inside. That's deconstruction ... You can only deconstruct what you love. Because you are doing it from the inside, with real intimacy ... You enter it.*

[ ]

The OB guides my hand inside our open patient so that my palm is pressed against uterus: smooth, warm, alive. She hands me a surgical instrument to help keep the uterus ajar, and I sweat and watch as she goes elbow deep into this woman, nodding to me at the baby's visible head as she pushes and pulls. I'm looking into a kind of portal, lush with shades of red, blue, purple. With one final, powerful movement,

she releases the baby from its shelter, and we behold
a stunned, pale thing that is, for a moment, still
and unrealizing. Baby soon cries out—ugly, sweet,
and writhing.

[   ]

It's 5 a.m., and I'm looking into the eyes of a bundled
newborn babe who, it seems to me, must be queer as
sunlight seeking every empty space. Good morning,
first morning, sweet babe. I have books heavier than
you. I've known flowers older than you, strange
bundle that you are. Most others have gone to bed,
but here we are—basking in the afterwardness of the
day's events, like two sparrows studying the forest,
picking broken branches after a storm.

[   ]

I hope you know, always, the pleasures of hot coffee,
alone at sunrise, then again at noon. Of the touch of a
foot at night. Of friendship, forsaken and unforsaken.
Of rose portraits, of still life and fruit, of messy desks,

your own desk. Of devotion, to yourself and
otherwise. Of the arbitrary that feels like the uncanny
that feels like your possibility. Of colour and of line.
Of your body on the floor, like a gesture to elsewhere
and right here, like ecstasy. I hope you know that
something in you will be reborn, several times over,
and today, for the first time
when you emerged like an aria, addressing all of us,
like a dream
and we thought:
what if we did everything in the other's stead.

[   ]

If you study what makes something beautiful, are you
closer to knowing what beauty is? Because I know the
ocean can be beautiful, its waves, how the water and
the wind, without looking, without touching, without
naming each other, form seven waves at seven o'clock,
waves that crash with and without purpose into the
shore, tied to and free from temporality, like ghosts.

[   ]

I'm not getting it right; I'm not writing it as it is—the full sensorium that is beauty that is the ocean that is the wind. Maybe, then, beauty is where language fails, where language must give itself over to something else, to an embodiment that cannot be held by a slim treatise of words. But are beauty's whereabouts beauty itself? If I have led you to the place of beauty, is it meaning enough?

[   ]

And yet. Against these odds, there is language and poetry as beautiful as ocean or flower, there have been writings so particular, so impossibly beautiful. Could it be that it's that moment of touch—that *kingdom of touching*—where the finitude of language touches the transcendent, maybe that place I want to know better, and it's not a question of beauty at all, but a journey to coordinates where the writing in the air creates a real, material elsewhere.

[   ]

I leave the country for clinical rotations abroad and promise to write you. The letters prove to be deeply performative, but writing them is perhaps some of the roundest pleasure I've felt. Round in the manner of Anne Carson, who writes:

> *desires as round as peaches*
> *bloom in me all night, I no longer*
> *gather what falls.*

[ ]

I have been gathering what falls for months, for years, in that search for beauty, but I write to you like someone unravelling, because this time I am what's falling, and I see no reason to gather myself.

[ ]

An excerpt from the letters:

I could describe the poles of my desire by recounting the coast of Portugal, the coast of Ireland.

The former is an ocean so brashly blue, so brightly blue, so brazen in its blueness, that no person could look away, no person could allow anything other than that blue in their whole frame of looking. Hundreds of us face the water, our backs to the beach, laughing and screaming and coughing as huge, unrelenting waves wash over us, pull us away and in, then nudge us back and upright. It's so salty that every orifice—eye, mouth, nose—burns like hell, but it's worth it and it's perfect and I am small but I am free.

The Irish beach, meanwhile, is overcast, windy, remote. I sit quiet and bundled by the water, writing, completely alone, drawing ellipses wherever I please, unfinished sentences and imprecise words filling my notebooks like pressed flowers, recognized finally for their wildness, known finally as precious and vital.

[   ]

Other times, I write to you, pleading: *I want you to know I am filled with an exquisite longing—I'm wavering between several hundred small islands, I feel like a shuddering archipelago, I don't want a boat or a rope, I'm willing you to fill your cupped hands with water.* Your

responses are shorter, less pleading. Your words feel
delicate, their mutability both excites and calms me.

[   ]

Have I been making the argument that beauty can be
found in the lover's discourse, in dialogues of desire,
dialogues on love? But so much of that discourse, I now
realize, is asking each other the same questions,
studying, together, the same ideas by new methods of
touch, new translations of I-want-you, I-love-you. At
least, this has been my experience. And sometimes, in
the space between question and answer, we escape, for
a moment, the hierarchies and taxonomies that regulate
our thoughts and our lives. Sometimes we reach the
alleged fulcrum, there was never anything there, and
together we're suspended in a great wisp of life.

[   ]

Beauty in repetition, then, or you and I asking each
other, in turns, why these handfuls of paper? I mean
Ocean Vuong's *handfuls of paper*; he says: *the world's on*

fire and here I am, obsessing over a handful of paper.
Perhaps the world's burning could be assuaged by
what's expressed in those handfuls of paper. Or perhaps
what assuages is the handfulness of the papers, how one
needs not a few poems but many, how one needs a great
many drafts, stacks of them, endless revisions for beauty.

[   ]

What of beauty as handfuls of paper, as handfuls of
paper that do not, that cannot, do what they have set
out to do; beauty as poems that are failures, poems
that are simply other versions of their failed selves,
each failing more than the last, each like a shout in
the night, unintelligible, intelligible, a particle of the
universe, but always splitting open, however small,
however painful.

[   ]

We start to see summer flowers, lavender especially, in
small bushels everywhere. One morning, we find a
field of it, *ostokhondoos*. We dissolve in an onrush of

fragrance, and we look at each other to say: sometimes, let's do away with subtlety.

[   ]

Lavender also lives by the entrance of the hospital—fresh and afloat in early-morning air. I'm drawn to its barely-bent posture, its playful purple. But if I stay with lavender for too long, I start to want it in abundance. Because I recognize each small gathering of lavender as synecdoche for umpteen fields of lavender. I'm not sure whether *synecdoche* is the right word here, but I don't know how else to say that lavender is enough, it can only stand in for more lavender, and the whole of lavender is just infinite lavender.

[   ]

Summer, I think, is not a season for palimpsests. You don't look for things concealed, for clues to the past or to the future, there is only the humidity that holds us in its idleness, its insistence upon languor, peeling the hair from the neck, pulling it high to the top of

the head, bare shoulders, warm berries in the hand,
lavender craning at the ankles, and then the gift of
rain, whose music reminds us of every return.

[   ]

A luxury! To lie next to each other, no need to conjure
each other through poem or prose. No need to waste
words on anything other than: here-is-another-way-
that-I-love-you, and where-should-we-go-to-lie-next?

[   ]

Us, here, flat on our backs, like rocks or remains,
is the beautiful thing I hold in my mind,
an artwork that's not abstraction.
We could make a habit of it,
the ritual of resting head into the earth,
arm hairs just inches from you; we're not the same,
but we're made of the same; eventually I roll into you,
the smell of your side like a salve. I pray it never causes
me pain to smell you, to remember you.

[   ]

What isn't fragile? Not the purple flower, not beauty, not the book on beauty, not the heavy summer that's always only brief, not even the place on the belly where you've been touched, where the flesh has hardly moved, has remained as it is, and yet belly becomes belly because it's been touched, cheek becomes cheek because it presses into belly, touched back in turn. And what's the point, really, note after note about how this is fragile, how that is fragile, how fragility is constitutive of our very existence as touching-feeling things. This note itself, language itself, most fragile of all. Why? I seem to return to the same revelations over and over, simple and clear as they are.

[   ]

All our essays and poems are made up of echoes and reconfigurations of each other. Do we return to the same ideas, the same refrains, by habit or by virtue of the thought itself, where some thoughts are essentially generous, new things to say each time?

[   ]

Another image that hasn't left me, that haunts me for
no agreeable reason, that I return to like a spectator
witnessing each time for the first time: it's a very early
morning at the hospital, surgery about to start, I sit by
the window facing the street and: a girl walks by with
bright orange hair, clearly dyed, carrying a giant green
plant, leafy, white flowers peeking behind the leaves,
or is it a separate bouquet, I can't really tell,
the inconvenience of desire flickers in me
and I describe her,
wondering what other than language
could fill the gulf between us.
She keeps walking and is gone,
but here I have my fragment.

[   ]

(I believe we've disavowed description for too long, as
though its gestures and its shapes, its associative
nature, its generous personality, how it comes to be
by way of some other person or art or thing, is not
original enough, not utterative enough.)

[   ]

I couldn't identify her flowers, our encounter was
too short, and so during that morning's surgery, and
most surgeries in the weeks thereafter, I embellish
the memory and reimagine the flowers so that they
could be: tulip/daisy/daffodil, *laleh/jhevra/narges*,
but it's too late, the chronic inaccuracy has taken
hold of me.

[ ]

Is it frustrating or freeing or both to imagine that we
might never truly articulate the meaning of anything,
that we only ever write in synonym, all our poems
somewhere slightly else, meaning as vagrant and open
as our own little bodies, no remedy for fragility, only
our ability to grapple, to reckon, and sometimes we
do it with grace or with gratefulness.

[ ]

Someone, a sort of friend from grad school, suggests
that I think of flowers during surgery because surgery
is "so masculine" and flowers are "the perfect

feminine antidote." I agree, as one so often does, with
the sneaking feeling that something has gone astray,
because at the moment of our exchange, I can't find
the words to say that his postulation is not quite right.

[   ]

Because I am taken instead by the strangeness of
flowers, a strangeness familiar and unfamiliar.
Flowers could be called queer, their style, their
manner of swaying in the half-light, dressing and
undressing, spread-eagle, leaning against each other,
exhaling, falling apart, coming back together,
dying then living. Yes, flowers have long been of
the realm of woman, whatever that might mean,
but I like flowers not for their softness or beauty, but
for the way they peer back at you—amused,
unflinching, curious, but still not too fussed with us.
Though their peering might, after all, be the displaced
centre of beauty.

[   ]

One surgeon speaks at length about the great standard of precision it takes to make a colostomy bag, how you mark the exact right spot, cut just so, pull with a measured tug, then suture in brisk fashion. But it was far more nonchalant and untidy from where I stood, on tiptoes, too stunned to feel queasy. Make a hole in the abdomen, reach for the intestine until it emerges from the belly, then sew it down onto skin so inside is continuous with outside. Another surgeon remarks that it looks just like a little rosebud: pink, round, pretty. Little stools slip out and you know it works. Secure the bag, stand back. A work of art, the surgeon says.

[ ]

As a medical student, I may have wasted too much time painting medicine as entirely awful and mundane. Before that, as a graduate student, I wasted more time taking art and medicine for granted as stable categories, trying to make use of their supposed sites of intersection. I projected an entire map, where binaries cross smoothly through each other, denying excess and complexity. I am trying now to observe, first, before anything else. This might be a more worthwhile effort. Instead of

forging or imagining clean, complete crossings, I might
feel, or take note of: where things touch.

[   ]

Where things touch: one home for beauty.

[   ]

To devote oneself to the study of beauty is to offer
footnotes to the universe for all the places and all the
moments that one observes beauty. I can no longer grab
beauty by her wrists and demand articulation or
meaning. I can only take account of where things touch.

[   ]

Solmaz Sharif writes: *I want a poetry of proximity, not
just by theme or figure, not just by metonymy or metaphor,
but by physical proximity by frame.* Sometimes I think I
know such a poetry by the muffled sounds of hearts in

my ears—lovers', patients'—by my wandering citations
lists, by the useful game of lifting a word from its house,
turning it over in my hands, placing it elsewhere to
name other things, seeing how it does, like a plant
carried from one patch of sunlight to another.

[   ]

Where things touch, or, E. M. Forster: *only connect.*

[   ]

We read *Howards End* in Modern British Literature.
I was eighteen and enraptured by my young professor.
I hoped that I, too, could someday speak like her
about literature, that I could make slow books seem
gripping, make complex ideas seem transparent, and
show so carefully that the pursuit of clarity is noble
and pleasurable. I felt that she never wasted words.

[   ]

In her class on *Howards End*, I saw the word *queer* on
a giant screen in an auditorium for the first time.

The slide's title: *Queer reconsidered as...*
The slide's text: *...the open mesh of possibilities, gaps,
overlaps, dissonances, and resonances, lapses and
excesses of meaning when the constituent elements
of anyone's gender, or anyone's sexuality, aren't made
(or can't be made) to signify monolithically.*

[   ]

Before that moment, I had encountered few things so
beautiful. Language was falling to pieces, and queer was
a fragment like a bird, crossing an unnameable chasm,
the inexpressible space between myself and myself.

[   ]

I recently read more from Sedgwick's *Tendencies*, and
she clarifies: *there are important senses in which "queer"
can signify only when attached to the first person* (only
connect). I remember wondering about my

professor's connection to queer; why did she care? I remember wondering whether my wondering was worrying for its assumption that she ought to spill into her work, that she was open. Now I might name such a spillover as beauty.

[   ]

Lately, learning to speak in the second person is the queer project that preoccuppies me most. When I write you, when I write to you, sometimes carelessly, sometimes with every intensity I have.

[   ]

A friend tells me about a writing course she's teaching that's mandatory for all first-year students in humanities programs. We reminisce about a similar course we took in our first year, where we learned that concision gets you closer to clarity, that *ooze* and *moist* and *leak* are unappealing words, that writing an entire essay with only one-syllable words is a useful exercise. We learned something about how short, small words can pierce, how simple, unassuming phrases can shatter you, how writing is editing, how writing is thinking, how to skin an essay and pare it down in spite of your attachments.

[   ]

Even back then, I wanted more than anything else to invoke beauty. But I believed in a beauty concerned with thick sentences, detailed ekphrasis, description as analysis, abundance as the most interesting aesthetics.

[   ]

In medicine, concision is also considered a crucial skill. Students are expected to "present a patient" and tell the patient's story to their supervising physician as efficiently as possible. Except nearly every body is moist; nearly every body oozes. And what a relief it might be, what a possible pleasure, to hear a patient's unadulterated version of events, to allow the story to seep through its own cracks.

[   ]

Though I can't discount the disgust that we, clinicians, feel at our pleasure, our practised efforts to repress it, and the inevitable contempt for the overly chatty patient, the anxiety of how-to-maneuver-to-my-next-question? And our shared delusion that the hospital is falling apart more quickly and more irreparably with every extra word they speak.

[   ]

There's satisfaction, I know, in editing and eliminating, but we deny ourselves the feeling of letting things spill over, of using an unseemly string of adjectives, each both closer to and farther from some original idea.

[   ]

I wonder if some things, like beauty, can only be known obliquely through language, but in the body, beauty is understood most acutely, most precisely.

[   ]

As Hélène Cixous puts it: *I, too, overflow; my desires have invented new desires, my body knows unheard-of songs. Time and again I, too, have felt so full of luminous torrents that I could burst—*

[   ]

I still feel the blood of my vessels get hot when I remember the look of horror and delight in your eyes when I said, out loud, what I wanted you to do next.

[   ]

Another practice of beauty: yielding and unyielding to you.

[   ]

You're interested in thinking more about what we're doing with—or what we're doing to—patriarchal relations. You ask: Can we write in a language outside of it? Can we touch in a language outside of it?

My response never changes: Yes. So often we are alienated from our bodies, from our sensuality, and yet one thing I know for sure is that some realizations of desire leave little in their wake other than bodies marvelling at the possibility of address.

[   ]

I can describe myself so that things become controlled, possible, the-next-rational-step. Other times, things come cascading out of my mouth in excess of everything that is. Sometimes, beauty is restraint. Other times, beauty is the fruit of that restraint: releasing to sensation after the wait, celebrating, freely and without shame, all the sensual details of our daily lives.

[   ]

Pain is one detail that is harder to celebrate. In the family medicine clinic, a lot of the pain that patients experience is attributed to different varieties of inflammation, which is understood as the body's innate response to injury or infection. Cells of the immune system travel to the site of injury and cause warmth, redness, swelling, and pain. At first, there is a moment of tension, or vasoconstriction, but then the vessels dilate, opening for a rush of blood. Vessel walls become permeable; new things get through and other things get out. Fluid accumulates and interrupts the smooth slope of substance or skin. Tissue becomes distorted, strange chemical mediators arrive at the interlude, and then there is pain.

[   ]

I interview a young patient about her chronic pain. I ask her to rate the severity of her pain on a scale of 1 to 10 in various domains of how it affects her life. She responds "10" to nearly every prompt. We get to talking and I learn that the pain began, in its mildest form, in the midst of a breakup nearly half a decade ago. A breakup that left her, she says, in pieces. These days, the pain is usually better in the mornings and starts to get worse at night.

[   ]

I can return again to Solmaz Sharif's poem "Beauty,"
the part that goes:

Most mornings
No, not morning
Morning I am still new
Still possible, I'm still possibly

[ ]

How to capture the feeling of *possibly*? How to make
it last? But I get ahead of myself, this patient never
asked for the feeling of morning in any tablet or vial.

[ ]

I want to remember these early days of my training,
when I don't know the medical world as normal,
when its investments in ideology are more obvious,
when poeticizing medicine seems like an attainable
intervention, when my clinical knowledge is so sorely
limited that I can't imagine any reasonable answer to

experiences of pain. I can only offer silences, questions, poems. So I ask about breakups, I ask about grief.

[   ]

Frida Kahlo's painting *La Columna Rota* is a self-portrait of a column ripping through her body, shooting up where her spine should be, tearing her in half. A corset-like cast restrains her body and tries to keep her whole, but the spreading of herself is too powerful. Little tears fall from her eyes, and little nails puncture the surface of her skin. Her pain comes from everywhere and from nowhere. Her pain dislocates the Pangaea that she was, and the shards come together differently now.

[   ]

Beauty is awake here, in this painting. Some places, beauty sleeps. But *La Columna Rota* is where beauty's eyes are open, where beauty reaches its very border, where beauty shakes as though about to shatter, where beauty is our challenge. We cannot separate

beauty from the unendurable, it does not soften or
make pain palatable, it's not to be used for cruel or
paternalistic meaning-making; to know beauty, here,
is to know, at the very least, the cacophony of excess
and contradiction that is our lives.

[   ]

La Columna Rota is not a painting about mending or
curing. Kahlo looks at me unflinchingly—she dares
me to meet her gaze. She's not looking for empathy or
excavation—she doesn't want my OT, PT, MD. I can
only receive her in our estrangement. It would be
violence to mine her for something that connects us,
in order to love her or to care. As Virginia Woolf says
about the person in pain, Kahlo opens herself up to
me, or at me, or near me, *to be just held in solitude.*

[   ]

John Berger writes that *the impulse to paint comes neither
from observation nor from the soul, but from an encounter.*
Such encounters, he explains, require *the nerve to get close*

enough for a collaboration to start. And to go in close is to forget *convention, reputation, reasoning, hierarchies, and self.* Going in close presents risks of destabilization, for both painter and subject. But going in close is probably how any person might inhabit herself as fully human, as a citizen of vulnerability only, after all. What I read as Berger's suggestion that painters contend honestly with forces of encounter is a helpful model of engagement for elsewhere places, too: the clinic, the home.

[   ]

We find a place together, and the walls are as yellow as egg yolk or sunlight or the pupils of daisies. We're uncertain about such colour—is it warm or is it garish? Someone cites Maggie Nelson in *Bluets*: she paints her apartment a *yellow of utter rage*, and says, *later I learned that nearly all cultures have considered yellow one of, if not the least attractive of all colours.* Nonetheless, she paints everything with it, comes to hate it, and soon moves out. Yellow, for Nelson, is ultimately unbeautiful.

[   ]

Goethe on yellow: *in its highest purity it always carries with it the nature of brightness, and has a serene, gay, softly exciting character.* To this point, we are amenable. Alas, the man goes on: *it is, on the other hand, extremely liable to contamination, and produces a very disagreeable effect if it is sullied.* He asserts that by a *slight and scarcely perceptible change*, yellow becomes the colour of *ignominy and aversion.*

[   ]

We promptly go to the hardware store and buy $100 worth of white paint. But that night, as we lie together on our mattress on the floor, we are buoyant in our yellow kingdom. We list all the yellow things we consider beautiful, things other than the walls of Maggie Nelson's shitty apartment:
rice and saffron, turmeric
dawn: where light spills between the mountains
as through a sieve,
honey poured over cream over barbari,
a gold chain with names carved in its pendant,
a sunlight of no specific impulse,
playing in clear streams of water,

and you, glowing like alabaster
where I touch your skin with my skin.

[   ]

We return the white paint and dwell in yellow,
a corner of beauty that I determine to henceforth
always hold dear.

[   ]

To our yellow house, another ex, this time mine,
starts sending yellow letters. By which I mean, they
describe another yellow: my hands squeezing lemons,
every last drop, over so many meals we once shared,
over mint salads, yogourt, fish. Or *The Days of
Abandonment*, a book of theirs I never returned, with
its yellow title on a blue cover; they don't ask for the
book back, and instead appeal to the ethical
consequences of having read such a thing, accusing
me of reading with detachment; in other words: how
could you leave me, how could you leave me. One
letter includes a quote from the book: *Even if the*

relationship shatters and ends, it continues to act in
secret pathways, it doesn't die, it doesn't want to die.

[　]

They're beautiful letters, even the demands for love,
the painful visions of an unconsummated future, even
the nostalgia that seems at times like a disease.

[　]

I accept that our new home is haunted by past loves, that
our bodies have been known to others. I accept that even
though you and I imagine we live, to use Anne Boyer's
phrase, in *a communism of two*, really, it's an affair among
many, each new embrace touched by historical embraces,
each new disclosure in conversation with all the
secrets we've shared with other people, each intimacy
burning with its own specificity, but never in isolation
from intimacies come to pass, intimacies still passing.

[　]

I discard the letters. Although the way forward is not clear, it is the only manner of burying I know.

[   ]

In an essay on Barthes' The Neutral, I read: *Words, of course, do not simply vanish,* verba volant; *one cannot even take them back without adding to them, without saying more words.* And what a dangerous possibility, after all, to think we could forget or erase or destroy that which came before.

[   ]

I don't bury letters imagining erasure. On my bravest days, I want to bury letters the way you might bury seeds, slightly off-centre, with a flawed intuition. What grows, how it grows, crooked creature of beauty, capacious garden bed, all of these I imagine as a poetics, as a way out of repression, a way of expression, an alternative to a denial that waits, that makes its appearance at the most pivotal and inopportune moments,

showing up in the mundane, too, jostling you,
chipping away at you.

[   ]

And by poetics I mean the scholar Hamid Dabashi's
poetics: *an angular take on reality, an aquiline
protrusion into its claim to straightforwardness.* Poetics,
or the bird taking a tangent into elsewhere, or me, my
fragment beneath the earth, beauty as the richest
possible soil, beauty as food for becoming. Beauty is
not indulgence, beauty is our right.

[   ]

More from Solmaz Sharif's poem "Beauty":

*Cleaning out the sink drain
The melted cheese
The soggy muesli
My life can pass like this
Waiting for beauty*

[   ]

Months later, you leave me, only for a few days, but presumably it's over between us. It starts with an argument over some equivalent of cleaning or sink drains and the sharing of domestic labour. In our distance, I'm left to remember all the days before you. Days I spent with my own clogged drain, melted cheese, soggy muesli, stale almonds in my pockets, walking to the hospital in the dark morning, few friends, dirty floors, patients crying or bleeding.

[　]

How easy to say that this was it, this was all it was, my life, and that you, my love, you were the beauty I had been waiting for. But as Sharif goes on to say: *A life is a thing you have to start.* And there were many starts in my aloneness.

[　]

Before you, yes, I was more or less alone. I lived alone with my cat, alone with my jasmine in a pot, my pothos in a pot, my half-read books, my tiny table, my

floral bedspread, my old floors, my windows, my blue
bowl that I filled with oranges every week, unpeeling
one fruit each morning. These were the things that
allowed my life to start, habits at home that seemed at
the time like repetitions without a cause and without
meaning, but looking back, these were habits of
beauty, of pleasure, how I knew connection.

[   ]

You eventually return home, sit next to me. I reach
for your hand, put my head in your lap, and it
scarcely matters what we call it, but I'll call it our
first summer again:
you sitting under a tree,
looking out into the linen twilight,
me lying on your thighs,
eating watermelon with sticky lips,
kissing the grass in thanks
that there we were,
soft, sentient stones
of an enchanted night.

[   ]

I asked for beauty,
you showed up on my stoop.

[   ]

Facing homeward, our perpetual orientation. By any
limerence or language, all our returns seem to be
home, all our arrivals seem to be home. By home I
don't mean mother's lap or mother's land; I mean
where air is clear, fire is light, earth is delicious, and
our bodies are shores for the ocean. Where we
sacrifice the ineffable for love.

[   ]

I interview for residency programs, and they point out
that I list "imaginative" as one of my strengths in my
written application. Tell us more about that. I blank.
I don't have a thing to say. We sit in a brief silence,
and my mind, in a way that cannot be explained or
accounted for, remembers the ocean. A sliver of sunlight
escapes through the blinds behind my interviewers,

and I wish I could free that light into the sea, where
it would be free to play its games of reflection and
refraction into oblivion.

[   ]

It can be helpful to write in a manner that Mary
Ruefle describes as follows: *turn vase into a hat and
wear it (*your *body becomes an upside-down flower).*
To me, these instructions have always been an
assignment to allow the thing to catch the light,
to allow its rays to occupy small space, third space,
in me, to let in the mystery thus, to turn that which
is sincere into that which is play. To remark at
patterns, but rearrange where might be interesting.
Maybe this is what I meant when, in my application
for residency training, I called myself imaginative:
solicitude for rearrangement, for upside-down
flowers, looking at what's around me, discerning
beauty, and in the way of Sharon Olds, binding
myself to the earth.

[   ]

Lia, of Dionne Brand's novel *Love Enough*, describes beauty as *a combination of light and time*. Beauty weighs less than pain; it doesn't incinerate you or burn a hole through you. It is fleeting; it never stays long enough to damage you. I can only imagine, then, that beauty lives in the broken shard, both accumulative and alone, a brief polyphony that tips our upright bodies into the horizontal plane, spreading like sky.

[   ]

It was you who showed me this quote from Brand, taking pictures of pages with your phone, sending them to me where I was, interviewing several provinces away. It's the only way in: to bend toward beauty, to write into beauty, to know ourselves as embedded, bellies open like palms, making poems from pieces.

[   ]

At another interview, they ask me about my interest in "interdisciplinarity": what do physicians-in-training have to gain from reading poems or from looking at art? I offer some answers in earnest: the humanities can teach us how to better listen to and interpret people's stories, the humanities develop our skills of observation and analysis, they extend our imaginative potential, and perhaps in some cases move us to make connections between our patients' private lives and broader social and political structures. My interviewers nod, maybe moderately interested or partially convinced. Though I might just be reading, in their response, my own investment in or commitment to the matter.

[   ]

Because that evening, as I ride the subway home, reading Rumi—*the ocean pours through a jar, and you might say it swims inside the fish!*—all I know is that this particular poem and these particular words are words of beauty, and they fill me with joy. *The mystery gives peace to your longing and makes the road home, home.*

[   ]

What sort of joy? I feel opened, or elsewhere. It's not unlike lying in the grass, in *damavand*, warm nights, wondering, in no hurry, what keeps the stars apart. We might call this a *radical decentering*, which Elaine Scarry describes as one means by which beauty orients us toward justice. *It is not that we cease to stand at the center of the world, for we never stood there. It is that we cease to stand even at the center of our own world. We willingly cede our ground to the thing that stands before us.* In other words, in the presence of beauty, we are beside ourselves, the pull of self-interest loosens, and we feel called to the caretaking of beauty, and we act to *protect or perpetuate a fragment of beauty already in the world.*

[   ]

But what I need to make clear: beauty is not the object, not the face, not the landscape, not even the flower. Beauty is the co-constitution of human and flower; beauty is the engagement between text and text; beauty is the practices of a place that knows everything as connected, beauty is the excesses of queer, of strangeness, beauty is every tension and every shattering. So what Scarry describes as the effect of, or a response to, a beautiful thing is, to me, more accurately the beautiful thing itself. What interests me is not so much the perpetuation of beauty, not so much closed normativities of beauty. What interests me, what astonishes me, is beauty as the body changing shape, the body's visceral, affective, and aesthetic alchemy with all the matter that surrounds it.

[   ]

To that end, I consider fragments almost inherently beautiful. So I'm compelled toward that which remains, or what's left behind, or what's preserved, or broken, or things unfinished, things in isolation but still reaching, what couldn't be destroyed, what survives. And I slip between the urge to bring fragments together or let them apart.

[   ]

Sometimes when I look at you, sitting across the table, by the window,
reading, drinking coffee, I know that same feeling

of opening/adjacent for the way that the light marks
your border,
casting the sun across the lower half of your face
so your edges are jagged but lovely, like glass.

[   ]

Intimacy, too, can be that radical decentering. Stacey
D'Erasmo writes: *Intimacy as disturbance, a force that
wakes you up...snatches you out of yourself, brings a
liberating knowledge of the beyond, of the limits of the
self in a much bigger universe.*

[   ]

But intimacy is not always the sudden, waking force.
Sometimes intimacy is the slow, daily habit of love,
the rolling over of the body in bed, shifting the other
ever closer to the edge, the buying of two litres of
milk rather than one, washing their yellowing
undershirts, and the occasional intrusive thought of,
what if they die? What if today's the day, on their
bike ride home? For no other reason than by the

slight of a momentarily distracted driver, what if
they're just: gone? And I'm left waiting, waiting for
their touch, the touch that assures me I am here.

[　]

Such things—the washing of clothes, the sharing
of milk, breathing together through the night,
lighting a candle with another candle so you might
eat by a softer light—these are some of the
aesthetics of our lives. And I've learned so much
about care, the attentiveness it takes, the pleasure
it makes, by thinking about, by caring for
aesthetics. It's an epistolary practice, really, they
are like love letters to you:
the dill, a garnish for the eggs,
kissing the ear of all things,
reading bits out loud like:
perhaps one day you touch the young branch,
sharing it more than once,
forgetting it's been shared before,
an inconsequential forgetfulness.

[　]

Another example: the pomegranate around which we sit, cross-legged, sharing it with our red hands. How the peel clings to its seeds, how bloody the whole thing is, how sour it tastes and sweeter still—the pomegranate tree and its fruit, no need for excessive symbolism to make it beloved or essential.

[   ]

~~Paying, giving,~~ offering attention, sustained and wide, to pomegranate or otherwise, is loving, I think.

[   ]

Another place to attend to aesthetics: poetry. We learn, as English students, about the symbiotic relationship between the poem's form and content. It is important and second nature to look/listen carefully to all aspects of the literary apparatus of the text. How, in John Donne's poetry, the comma is absolutely significant: *And Death shall be no more, Death, thou shalt die!*

[   ]

Thinking about Donne's words, Professor Ashford, of Margaret Edson's play *W;t*, explains: *Nothing but a breath—a comma—separates life from life everlasting... It's a comma, a pause... Not insuperable barriers, not semicolons, just a comma.* (Another third space, that which separates life from life everlasting, or to wherever the comma gestures.)

[   ]

The form, the aesthetics of a work—how it's built, curve of letter, formations of text, whether block or column or circle, the sounds of words together, symbols or motifs that repeat (flower), moments of caesura, the last word upon which things rest—is meaning, is utterance, and all of it exceeds what the poem is "about." We take note of where things touch.

[   ]

A few years ago, less so because I was younger and more so because I was writing essays and theses of a certain kind as schoolwork, I'd read a poem at face value and

try to extract its "message." I would render the poem a
cadaver, dissecting and exploiting its many parts for
tools to advance my project, discarding or denying
elements that contradicted or confused me. I imagined
a false binary between form and content, suffocating
the intimate, insoluble relationship of form and content,
the total continuum, the peel clinging to the seeds.

[   ]

These days, I feel that, more often than not, meaning
slowly emerges from a reading that allows the thing
to remain as itself—whole, having a life beyond my
contact with it.

[   ]

Something, too, about how the poem makes itself with
your lips, how your mouth forms an O. In a way, you
are the poem—or maybe you and the poem are kissing.

[   ]

I think of the I in writing as a feminist gesture—i.e., my
writings are inextricably tied to my particular body,
my political self; moreover, I'm accountable to what I
write. I wonder, though, if when I say "I" in a poem—
I paint flowers so they will not die—really, I mean "O." The
O of or, of oh, of of. O, the circle, the shape of a mouth.

[   ]

Your mouth, in particular, is the mouth I imagine
speaking the poem. It is your shape whose borders
give way to the im/material that is poetry, the shaking
fragment that is the poem.

[   ]

Suppose we allow I its relief, let I become O: your
mouth's shape. What, then, becomes of me when I is
like a synonym for the shape of your mouth? Is it my
doing or my undoing? (Everything likes to follow
from this principle:) Both.

[   ]

You know, I'd trade my youth for this: to write a few poems of you, fewer than five even. To be sure, I'd trade my youth for less—even just for knowing the L-shape your shoulder makes with your neck. Not to say that youth is somehow the most precious, and not to say that poems of you, your body's corners, your arms, are not the most precious. Because they are.

[   ]

This is what beauty is: the most precious but also not the most precious, many planes of meaning at once, the ubiquitous overlapping with the singular, no critical point but many kinds of caress, a foothold, a freefall, nothing and everything at stake. In other words, a poem.

[   ]

To say beauty is a poem is to say that beauty is both inside analysis and outside analysis. To say beauty is a poem is not to say that beauty is not material, not the everyday.

[   ]

Because many things are poems: the DSM, the afternoon, another afternoon when I read *Little Things* with a patient, not just the text itself but also our encounter—the pile of things swept up after a vase falls: glass, petal, debris, each piece like a stanza— when my supervising physician called on me, rather cruelly, for an answer that I couldn't quite remember, the angry tears I struggled to hold back. Poems as ongoing, collective projects, as ineffaceable but malleable, as always at the cusp of possibility. A poem is something to think deeply about, its construction filled with knowledge about the site of its emergence.

[　]

Regarding most things as poetry is not my romance with the world—studying poems is rigorous business. Though rigour and romance need not be different modes.

[　]

My teacher Daniel Coleman writes about Paul Ricoeur's strategies of interpretation. There are the *hermeneutics of suspicion*, where the object/text is understood *as an illusion or disguise which must be stripped away* as *the text is unaware of its own motivations or contents, and the reader needs to discover what it is that exists behind the text's lack of self-awareness.*

There are also the *hermeneutics of affirmation*, wherein *the process of reading or interpretation involves the realization or recollection of revelation's depth of meaning. The text is to be venerated, appreciated, and analyzed for its truth and beauty.* We need them together, Coleman offers, to more reasonably do this work of reading, writing, teaching, and healing.

[   ]

Reading, we might also remember, is a kind of ecological activity. Not just because wherever we read, and our particular situatedness, affects how we read: café or bedroom, aloud or silent, the city in which we read, the country in which we read, whether we hear sounds from the street, the way we sit, our embodiment, the weather, the climate, and so on. Not just because the materiality of what we read alters how we read: the feel of the printed page, new

book or old book, stolen or borrowed, computer
or hardcover.

[   ]

Reading is ecological for what it does to our ties to that
which lies around us: what and how we see when we
look up from the page. A hermeneutics of affirmation
for receptivity, for curiosity, for awe toward the beauty
of all the human, animal, and mineral worlds. And a
hermeneutics of suspicion to learn skills for discerning
all that threatens those worlds.

[   ]

Physicians, meanwhile, often seem to do away with both
postures in our institutional environments. But I should
speak for myself: on many a long stretch, I have allowed
both to get away from me—or have been made to let
go of both, an imperative to getting by. What happens
when the whole of hermeneutics slips away? Something
in the body, I think: a shrinking, an agitation, whatever
feels like the opposite of expansion. And in the hospital,

no less—where we are to do, ostensibly, the work of care, where our repressions as a human species come to bear violently on our bodies, where we attend, pretty much categorically, to the material consequences of our political systems.

[   ]

Maybe the search for beauty has just been my circular flight around one simple desire: to incorporate many more kinds of knowing into the work that I/we do as caregivers and caretakers of people, texts, other creatures.

[   ]

A quick note: although hermeneutics is like interpretation, it's more than just that—I suggest a hermeneutics that knows: *in place of a hermeneutics we need an erotics of art.* A hermeneutics that lets you deliver and be delivered by a text; a hermeneutics that can be *a hymn to sensual reality*;

a hermeneutics that can be felt in the chest or
belly or groin.

[   ]

Because even as I ask myself to linger in the empty
space of this page, or the space between each word
and the meaning to which it gestures, or the wide
breath of the wind that carries us—even as I imagine
the in-between, the empty space, I know that the
flesh, the stuff of it, is where I want to live.

[   ]

One final bit of beauty: the story of the bird called
Homa. She's said to never alight on the ground—she
lives her life flying so high above the earth that, to us,
she's invisible. From time to time, her shadow passes
over us, and we can gather its stillness. I don't know.
Is her shadow beauty? Is she herself—the bird—
beauty? Or maybe it's those fragments of stillness
we're given, fragments we might carry or curate, give

away and exchange. We wait for beauty, but beauty flies over us all the while, free. Beauty articulates herself in her own language.

[   ]

Shadows, sediment, wind, lullabies—these, I believe, are matters of love.

[   ]

You know, despite everything I've said, I'm wary of wasting words on love. By which I mean, I have already written and rewritten letters of love to you in great repetition; by which I mean, I've repeated myself with negligible variation, but I've still been sincere, and you continue to listen and to care. When did our misdemeanours, our every encounter like a rupture in my life, begin to feel normal? Love has been our slow oscillation between the feeling of wrong, the feeling of right, a boredom, a quiet, a light.

[   ]

By way of habit, we compile what you've called our
own *glossary of touch*. Our routines, knowing how you
wash your body, the little pile of socks on the floor,
the way you always prefer to drink from one mug and
not another, the walks we take, the silence after the
fight like the silence after the rain—these habits of
intimacy are among the few freedoms we can offer
each other.

[ ]

Kiarostami, whose films I would never describe as
cynical, says in an interview: *love is misunderstanding*.
And we might still wonder whether this is indeed a
cynical proposition, that we only love what we don't
understand, and once we do understand, the love
ends. In this case, *love is an illusion* as we project our
interpretations, insist upon them, fall in love with
them, and then recoil as they shatter.

[ ]

At the same time, however, misunderstanding is not
the antithesis of understanding, not the opposite. It's

a few degrees away, somewhere in-between, off-kilter, *an angular take on reality, an aquiline protrusion into straightforwardness.* The *mis* of *misunderstanding* has its roots in divergent, astray, diverse, various. Misunderstanding as proliferative, love as several. Or maybe *miss*-understanding: a longing for understanding, a posture toward understanding, a desire, a commitment, a queerness.

[   ]

But I suppose I learned this from you first,
that love is a curiosity
that every word we utter is a question
that when you move your body
into the space of my body
my skin your walls, my voice your roof
your limbs ask my limbs
can this be our home.

[   ]

Notes and Acknowledgements

The following is a list of works cited: *Beauty* by Solmaz Sharif; *Close-up* by Abbas Kiarostami; *Body Tracks* by Ana Mendieta; *In Search Of* by Sohrab Sepehri; *To look at the sea is to become what one is* by Etel Adnan; *Orientalism* by Edward Said; *On Beauty* by Elaine Scarry; *The Red Poppy* by Louise Glück; *Mend Piece* by Yoko Ono; *Towards a Poetics of the Whole Fragment* by Ann Lauterbach; *Silueta Series* by Ana Mendieta; *Gravity and Grace* by Simone Weil; *Because it is Beautiful* by Rita Felski; *Of Grammatology* by Jacques Derrida and translated by Gayatri Chakravorty Spivak; *The Wind Will Carry Us* by Forough Farokhzad; *Elegy* by Aracelis Girmay; *Plainwater: Essays and Poetry* by Anne Carson; *A Poetry of Proximity* by Solmaz Sharif; *Howards End* by E. M. Forster; *Tendencies* by Eve Sedgwick; *Laugh of the Medusa* by Hélène Cisoux; *La Columna Rota* by Frida Kahlo; *The Waves* by Virginia Woolf; *Steps Towards a Small Theory of the Visible* by John Berger; *Bluets* by Maggie Nelson; *Theory of Colours* by Johann Wolfgang Goethe; *The Days of Abandonment* by Elena Ferrante; *The Professor's Desire: On Roland Barthes's The Neutral* by Anca Parvulescu; *The World Is My Home: A Hamid Dabashi Reader* edited by Andrew Davison; *Short Lecture on the*

Nature of Things by Mary Ruefle; *Little Things*, by Sharon Olds; *Love Enough* by Dionne Brand; *The Road Home* by Rumi; *The Art of Intimacy*, by Stacey D'Erasmo; *W;t* by Margaret Edson; *In Bed With The Word* by Daniel Coleman; *Against Interpretation* by Susan Sontag; Interview with Abbas Kiarostami by *Criterion*; Interview with Anne Boyer by *Mythos*; Interview with Ocean Vuong by *The Well & Often Reader*; Interview with Forough Farrokhzad, source unknown.

Thank you, to all my dear friends, who sat with me, listened to me, read my work, and believed it could be possible, to all my teachers, especially my parents, and my little brother too, to Meg Storey for her kind and careful editing, to Jay and Hazel Millar, whose support has meant so much, to Metonymy Press, whose GBLU judges offered generous and exacting comments to an early draft of this book, and to all the writers and artists before me whose beautiful works I'll be writing back to all my life.

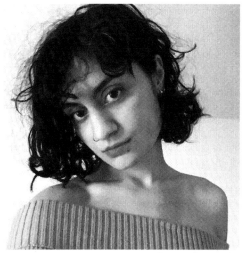

photo: Padina Bondar

Bahar Orang is a writer and physician-in-training living in Toronto. Her writing has been published in such places as *GUTS, Hamilton Arts & Letters, CMAJ,* and *Ars Medica. Where Things Touch: A Meditation on Beauty* is her first book.

Essais Series

Drawing on the Old and Middle French definitions of *essai*, meaning first "trial" and then "attempt," and from which the English word "essay" emerges, the works in the Essais Series challenge traditional forms and styles of cultural enquiry. The Essais Series is committed to publishing works concerned with justice, equity, and diversity. It supports texts that draw on seemingly intractable questions, to ask them anew and to elaborate these questions. The books in the Essais Series are forms of vital generosity; they invite attention to a necessary reconsideration of culture, society, politics and experience.

Titles in the Essais Series:

Her Paraphernalia: On Motherlines, Sex, Blood, Loss & Selfies
by Margaret Christakos (2016)

Notes from a Feminist Killjoy: Essays on Everyday Life
by Erin Wunker (2016)

Blank: Essays and Interviews
by M. NourbeSe Philip (2017)

My Conversations with Canadians
by Lee Maracle (2017)

Dear Current Occupant
by Chelene Knight (2018)

Refuse: CanLit in Ruins
co-edited by Hannah McGregor, Julie Rak,
and Erin Wunker (2018)

Before I Was a Critic I Was a Human Being
by Amy Fung (2019)

Disquieting: Essays on Silence
by Cynthia Cruz (2019)

The Nothing that Is: Essays on Art, Literature and Being
by Johanna Skibsrub (2019)

Where Things Touch: A Meditation on Beauty
by Bahar Orang (2020)

For more information and to order visit bookhugpress.ca

COLOPHON

Manufactured as the first edition of
Where Things Touch: A Meditation on Beauty
in the spring of 2020 by Book*hug Press

Edited for the press by Meg Storey
Copy edited by Stuart Ross
Type + design by Ingrid Paulson

bookhugpress.ca